意拳

Yiquan
and the Nature of Energy

Number One in the Nature of Energy Series

by Fong Ha

Revised and Updated

Summerhouse Publications
Berkeley, California
2019

ISBN: 978-0-578-40273-4

Summerhouse Publications is an imprint of BrightCityBooks, www.brightcitybooks.com.

Yiquan and the Nature of Energy is the first in a series of perspectives on the internal martial arts. Upcoming publications in the series will include: *The Essence of Taijiquan, Yijinjing and the Nature of Energy*, and *A Guide to the Taiji Ruler*. Additional titles will be announced in future issues.

Introduction

Just as the rosebud contains within it the innate form of the perfect flower, so do we all contain within ourselves the innate forms of our own perfection.

Under the proper conditions of sun, water, and nutrients, the bud unfolds to reveal the rose. Likewise, the simple practice of *Yiquan*[1], literally "intention practice," helps us break through a lifetime of old habits and programmed patterns of posture and movement, allowing what is essential in us — physically, mentally, and spiritually — to naturally unfold.

Yiquan incorporates physical and mental training into one simple system that requires no special equipment or skills. While it is a martial art, it is much, much more. It is a complete system of physical and mental cultivation that provides benefits for all. Anyone can learn and practice *Yiquan*, young or old,

1 Please refer to the glossary starting on page 39 for more about all terms and names.

ill or healthy. Performed a few minutes every day, this elegant and refined system for self-cultivation will develop your *qi* — your vital or internal energy — and focus your consciousness, or intention — your *yi* — for enhanced health and vitality, reduced stress, improved concentration, creativity and productivity, and greater peace of mind. This volume is intended to be a systematic, step-by-step guide to *Yiquan*.

"Avail yourself of the force of the universe, and bring your instinctive ability into full play." These are the words of Wang Xiangzhai, founder of the *Yiquan* system, my grand-teacher. Wang Xiangzhai was born in Hebei Province in China in 1885. In poor health as a child, he began studying *Xingyiquan* or "form & mind practice" with Master Kyo Yun-Shen. Though *Xingyiquan* is a martial art, Wang's original intent, like that of so many today, was to improve his health and realize his full potential. And like so many who begin the practice of the martial arts for health, Wang became devoted to his study, improving his health and along the way also becoming an accomplished martial artist.

As an adult, Wang traveled throughout China, seeking out and learning from the masters of a variety of different styles and systems, and by the time he was 30, had become one of China's foremost martial arts masters himself.

It was while teaching martial arts to Army cadets in Shanghai in the early 1920s that Wang had a key insight into the nature of human potential, and turned his attention once again to the realm of health. Wang realized most students paid too much attention to specific postures and patterns of movement, but neglected training their minds and spirits. Their movements may have been swift and powerful, he observed, but their movements were nonetheless "empty," and not as effective as they could be. Moreover, such physical training devoid of mental and spiritual training, Wang felt, created imbalances that could lead to illness and injury, if not psychosis. It was only the mind, or consciousness if you will, trained and refined and focused, that could fill the emptiness Wang saw in his students' movements, and correct the imbalances.

Wang thus set out to eliminate from his *Gongfu* (a general term for various styles of Chinese martial arts) anything that wasn't essential, anything that might interfere with his ability to respond naturally to whatever life might throw his way, be it aggression, disease, injury. The result of that process of synthesis and refinement was *Yiquan*. It became known as the "style of no style," a nicely ambiguous description that captures some of the quirky *Daoist* worldview that informs the practice.

"The goal of *Yiquan*," Wang said, "is to concentrate the spirit and stabilize the mind. Find the natural, inborn abilities."

While his system was popularly dubbed "*Dachengquan*" or "great achievement system," Wang thought that was a bit too grandiose, and preferred to call it simply *Yiquan*, "intention practice," to emphasize the importance of the mind in his art. Thus *Yiquan's* simplicity and emphasis on awareness, rather than complicated technique. Of course these insights, developed within the context of the martial arts, are applicable to all aspects of life.

I encountered *Yiquan* first-hand back in 1971, when I was visiting in Hong Kong and met one of Wang's students, Mr. Han Xingyuan. By then, Wang had died, and Han had grown to become well-known as an *Yiquan* master, martial artist, and healer.

By the time I met Han *Sifu* (*"Sifu"* is a title for an honored teacher, a.k.a. *"Shifu"*), I had been practicing the martial arts for more than 30 years, most of my life. I'd always been naturally athletic, strong and quick; these natural abilities combined with decades of training made me, I thought, a fairly formidable martial artist.

I had first been exposed to the martial arts as a little boy in Macau, where my father, a building contractor, had moved the family from Hong Kong temporarily to work on a construction project. I had a distant uncle in Macau, also named Ha, schooled in the Shaolin tradition, who was a rather well-known martial arts master, and my father encouraged me to study with him. However, I was very young, and I suppose I had a bit of a rebellious streak; I wasn't a particularly devoted student, in other words.

By the time our family returned to Hong Kong, the war had started and Hong Kong was under Japanese occupation, which didn't by any means help ease my natural tendencies toward rebelliousness, nor did the resumption of British occupation when the war ended. But I was much too young back then to know clearly what I was rebelling against, and so my rebellion expressed itself in the usual ways, including a rather pronounced dislike for school.

Rather than spend any more time than necessary on my homework, I devoted myself to reading comic books about martial arts masters like Yang Luchan, founder of the Yang style of *Taijiquan* we practice today. In the comics, Yang possessed the superhuman skills any good superhero must have, which he put to good effect as a champion of justice, defending the poor and oppressed, a sort of cross between Robin Hood and Superman, I suppose. Naturally, I fell in love at least with the *idea* of *Taiji*. The problem was, the only *Taiji* I saw in my neighborhood in Hong Kong at the time seemed to be practiced in parks by old people who spent quite a lot of their time standing around smoking. This wasn't my idea of rising up against the oppressor and fighting for justice.

Then one morning in 1953, as I was riding the train from my home to school, sitting by the window on the car's second level, I noticed a sign on a building directly across from me announcing *Taiji* in the style of Yang Chengfu, Yang Luchan's grandson. I was intrigued, but I rode past that building many times before I finally worked up the nerve to get off the train and go knock on the door.

I still remember vividly when Dong Yingjie (a.k.a. Tung Ying-chieh) answered. He was an old man by then, very tall and thin, with a shaved head. Behind him on a wall I could see some beautiful calligraphy, the characters for *qi* and *shen*, which I learned later he'd done. Not only was he a martial arts master, he was a remarkable calligrapher and scholar, a combination of skills that aren't uncommon, I've noticed, among those devoted to the practice of *Taijiquan* and related disciplines. I told him I wanted to learn *Taijiquan*. "Come in, come in," he said. I was immediately captured by his charisma, his kindness, and openness.

Until I moved to the U.S. in 1957 to attend college and then graduate school, I'd ride the train from school each evening and get off to study with Dong *Sifu*. I was very fortunate that he was my first *Taijiquan* teacher. His relationship with me was almost like that of a grandfather teaching his grandson.

In the U.S., I continued my practice, and as time and finances allowed, I returned to Hong Kong, and then later to mainland China, after China opened its doors a bit more widely, to meet and work with martial arts masters from a variety of schools and disciplines. This sort of intellectual commerce is the best way I know of to hone your own skills, and I believe that exposure to different styles, different ways of doing things, and different ideas and personalities helps you keep an open mind about your own practice.

These encounters would usually involve plenty of conversation, plenty of good food, and eventually some sort of "push-hands" practice. I'll have more to say in later volumes of this series about push-hands, but briefly, it's a two-person exercise that is an essential part of virtually all internal martial arts, that is, the martial arts that focus on the development of *yi* and *qi*, rather than on external forms.

In practice, push-hands can range from the gentlest sort of contact in which the two players try to sense, interpret, and respond to another's energy, to something close to outright freestyle combat, but always, push-hands is a special sort of "collaborative combat," in which the intention is not to harm or defeat your partner, but rather to help him or her develop his or her own skills, just as your partner helps you develop yours.

As I said, by the time I met Han *Sifu*, I thought of myself as a reasonably accomplished martial artist, but after pushing hands with Han for only a few minutes, I realized he was one of the finest martial artists I'd ever had the pleasure of encountering. His movements were fast, powerful, and precise. And what truly amazed me was how he always seemed to know what I was going to do before I did it. He seemed to be reading my mind, or more precisely, I would realize later, he was reading my intention, and in that split-second gap between my intention to act and the act itself, Han *Sifu* usually managed to position himself to respond appropriately. He was a very tricky opponent, in other words.

More amazing was Han's basic practice, an odd sort of standing meditation called *zhanzhuang* (*zhan*: stand, *zhuang*: pillar or foundation), which, I soon learned, is the heart and soul of *Yiquan* practice, and the main theme of this book. This isn't to say that Han didn't also diligently practice other, more obviously martial techniques, but these were few and deceptively simple, and all were practiced within the context of, and informed by *zhanzhuang* and by a certain attitude, which one might think of as the "*Yiquan* way."

What do I mean by the "*Yiquan* way"? Han was a descendant of a family deeply rooted in the internal martial arts tradition. He was already a master of *Baguazhang* and *Xingyiquan* by the time he met Wang Xiangzhai and became his student. And then like his teacher, Han *Sifu* proceeded to strip his practice to the bare essentials. At first glance, Han's system seemed much too simple, so simple in fact it seemed absurd that Han could have developed his extraordinary powers this way.

But this was the essence of the *Yiquan* way. Through these deceptively simple practices, we integrate the mind with the body, we develop *qi*, we learn to focus our intention more precisely, and we strip our reflexive responses of all the excess baggage of learned techniques, preconceived notions, or unconscious habits of carriage, behavior, and self-armoring picked up over a lifetime of hard knocks.

Yiquan doesn't emphasize tradition; the focus is on how to get results. How you feel is the important thing, not the perfect imitation of techniques learned from this or that master. *Yiquan* teaches the principle of returning to your own nature, of becoming your own master.

Through this practice, then, we allow our natural responses to whatever life sends our way to surface; in this, the ideas underlying *Yiquan* are very similar to those of *Daoism* and *Zen*. *Yiquan* helps us find the physical correlate to what in *Daoism* is called the *Dao* or "way," that is the natural, appropriate response or course of action that is in harmony with all around us.

The practice, and the physical and spiritual insights it offers, provides a firm center in a changeable world in which we are constantly bombarded with received ideas and ways of acting and being. Thus through

8

the martial art of *Yiquan*, we can physically confirm and reinforce the essence of a life philosophy and spiritual path. Both Wang and Han understood this; they viewed *Yiquan* as a way of transforming the self, and hoped it would transform society as well.

I found all of this to be very heady stuff, and soon after I met Han *Sifu*, I arranged for him to come to the U.S. to live with me for a time so my students and I could learn more from him.

Like most of Wang's students, Han *Sifu* was very open about his practice and always willing to share his knowledge, unlike masters from many other — perhaps most other — disciplines, who can be rather secretive. Wang himself felt that secretiveness was bad for the martial arts; he felt that the only way the arts could evolve, and with them the practitioners, was through openness and a mutual exchange of ideas. He thought the martial arts in particular were a great way of learning and sharing together, so he would share his insights with anyone who sought him out. Han thus epitomized Wang's ideals in his own practice and life.

Han lived and practiced with my students and me during the summers of 1976 and 1977. His teachings transformed my practice and approach to the martial arts; I began to concentrate less on external forms and techniques, and more on the *neigong*, that is the cultivation of our innate abilities and potential. Sadly, Master Han died two years after his second visit.

However, I was fortunate to meet another highly accomplished individual soon after, Cai Songfang of

Shanghai and Canton. Cai *Sifu* is one of China's most renowned *Qigong* masters. Though not a student of Wang, he had arrived at a way of practice and a philosophy of the martial arts that was very similar to those of *Yiquan*. Like Wang and Han, Cai had stripped his practice to the bare essentials, and like them, he put great emphasis on the role of a highly trained and focused consciousness in health, the martial arts, and all of life.

And like Han *Sifu*, Master Cai was also capable of "reading" an opponent's intention, then acting with precision and swiftness to anticipate and counter whatever his opponent was going to do. Moreover, Cai *Sifu* also seemed able to "read" my intentions from a distance. And not only that, he could respond at a distance, projecting what at first glance seemed a mysterious force across several yards to affect me. These weren't exactly blows from a distance, but rather odd, somewhat uncomfortable sensations of being pushed or having my centerline impinged upon.

This so-called "empty force" (*kongjing*) is the stuff of martial arts legend, and the stuff of every martial artist's dreams, that is to be able to affect or even "strike" an opponent from a distance. As a child in Hong Kong, I devoured stories about heroes who possessed this ability (in the stories, they could also usually walk on water, fly, and perform other amazing feats). While I was quite devoted to these tales, I doubted that empty force was more than legend, any more than the flying and all the other stuff, until I was on the receiving end of Cai *Sifu*'s own empty force. But I should say here that while many of Cai's students and others have developed the ability to use empty force, I think it's a mistake to view this as the final goal of *Yiquan* practice, as it becomes for many; I think this can be a digression from the true spirit of *Yiquan*, and I have more to say about this below.

Master Cai is also a very devout Buddhist and true humanitarian. For him, practice in the martial arts is just that, a *practice*. For him, it is simply a way of achieving self-realization and the development of one's potential — physical, mental, and spiritual. His great achievements in *Gongfu* are almost something of a "by product" of his pursuit of higher consciousness. He is also involved with a number of research projects and hospitals in China as a teacher and healer, conducting classes for patients to teach them how to develop their own *qi* for self-healing.

We became great friends almost immediately. Like Han *Sifu* had been, Master Cai is open about his practice and eager to share. He also has a great sense of humor. Fortunately, he has been able to come to the U.S. to live with me on two occasions, during which my students and I learned much from him. The program outlined here is a synthesis of Wang's *Yiquan* as it evolved through the work and insights of masters Han and Cai. ∎

A Few Concepts

Yiquan

Yiquan developed within a rich system of martial and healing arts, loosely classified as "internal" arts, that is disciplines that emphasize mental cultivation and cultivation of internal energy or *qi* over purely physical development. That's not to say these internal arts, *Yiquan* included, don't include physical training. But the emphasis, again, is on the consciousness, spirit, and *qi*, in contrast with external arts such as *Karate* or *Gongfu*, which emphasize training in speed, strength and techniques. Of course, practitioners of both the external and internal arts find common ground at the highest levels as they all strive for full integration of the mental, physical, and spiritual aspects of optimal performance; they simply go at this development from different directions.

More significant, perhaps, are the differences in the motivations of those who take up internal or external martial arts; whereas most who are attracted to the external arts tend to be interested in self-defense or competition, or at least a good hard workout, those who take up one of the internal arts are often more interested in health, healing, or self-realization. But many practitioners of external arts also practice the internal arts as a supplement to their other training, and vice versa. Thus the internal and external arts are truly democratic.

Yiquan, "intention practice," is a form of *Qigong*, literally "energy practice." But *Yiquan* differs from other *Qigong* systems in the emphasis it places specifically on the role of the mind in the development of *qi*, in healing, and for that matter in the martial arts. *Yiquan* specifically develops concentration and mental focus, and integrates mental, physical, and even spiritual or psychic energies.

While *Yiquan* specifically is a relatively recent development in the evolution of the martial and healing arts, its roots can be found in concepts that evolved in China millennia ago, and thus informed the development of *Taijiquan, Xingyiquan, Baguazhang*, and similar disciplines. These concepts are now found in the healing arts and techniques for rejuvenation based on physical, mental, and spiritual balance, of following the *Dao* — the path or "way" of nature — and *qi* — or vital energy, life force, or breath.

This mingling of martial, spiritual, and health practices into one discipline makes plenty of sense when we consider that practices like *Taijiquan, Qigong* and similar disciplines, and certainly the "external arts," evolved in rather more rough-and-tumble times, when being able to hold your own in a knock-down-dragout was essential to being healthy, and when being able to fight and being healthy were intertwined with spiritual development, or certainly with living long enough and well enough in hard times to develop the mind and spirit.

Qi

These internal disciplines all have as their fundamental goal the cultivation and marshaling of *qi* — *ki* in Japanese, *prana* as it's called in India — for improved health, vitality, longevity, and at the highest levels of practice, enlightenment. *Qi* has been variously translated as "life force," "breath," "universal energy," or "human energy field," though none of these translations quite captures the true meaning of these terms. In truth, English doesn't contain an exactly equivalent concept.

Here in the West, we've always made a pretty clear distinction between the body and the mind, flesh and spirit. Granted, here in the West we have on occasion given lip service to the idea that exercise and sport might have moral, intellectual or even spiritual benefits — a sound mind in a sound body and all that — but the moral, spiritual or other such benefits of physical activity have always been seen as something of a byproduct, and certainly the public behavior of many of our best athletes, and even some martial artists, would suggest that such training could be bad for one's character, not helpful. The primary goal of the Western athlete has always been to get stronger, faster, tougher, and, if the athlete happens to be very good, also richer. If some other benefits having to do with the mind or spirit also follow, so much the better, but it's not as if athletes in the West typically hope to deliberately advance spiritually through the practice, say, of shooting hoops or running laps.

In Asia and India, on the other hand, that conceptual division between body and mind or between exercise and spiritual growth never occurred with all the certainty that characterizes the split in the West; indeed, in Asia and India, a balance between the spiritual and physical is seen as the key to health and longevity, while imbalances lead to disease.

Thus disciplines like *Yoga*, *Taijiquan* and related practices such as *Aikido* have evolved in Asia and India with the express purpose of using physical and

14

mental exercises together to unite mind and body, and through that discipline to develop the spirit along with physical health, restore or maintain balance in the body, and increase the *qi* or life force.

Most cultures seem to have some similar concept of a life force or life essence that can be cultivated for improved physical or spiritual health. Curiously, Western cultures presently don't, perhaps because of the way we divide mind from body. But it has been argued that at the dawn of Western civilization and even through the Middle Ages and up to the Enlightenment, the West also possessed such a concept, and that the light shown radiating from saints in early Christian paintings, for example, is in some ways a representation of high levels of this "life force" or spiritual power. The Classical Greek term *pneuma* — breath, wind, or spirit, from which we derive words such as, alas, pneumonia — may be as close an approximation of *qi* or *prana* as we have in Western thought, at least as it's used to refer to spirit.

Whether *qi* is truly a "substance" like blood or air, or a "force" like the bioelectrical activities taking place inside our bodies, is open to debate. Fritjof Capra, author of *Tao of Physics*, suggests that *qi* is neither a substance nor a force, but rather a useful concept to represent or describe a *system*:

> The concept of Ch'i, which played an important role in almost every Chinese school of natural philosophy, implies a thoroughly dynamic conception of reality. The word literally means "gas" or "ether" and was used in ancient

China to denote the vital breath or energy animating the cosmos. But, neither of these Western terms describes the concept adequately. Ch'i is not a substance, nor does it have the purely quantitative meaning of our scientific concept of energy. It is used in Chinese medicine in a very subtle way to describe the various patterns of flow and fluctuation in the human organism, as well as the continual exchanges between organism and environment. Ch'i does not refer to the flow of any particular substance but rather seems to represent the principle of flow as such, which, in the Chinese view, is always cyclical.

It's an interesting idea, and one might even argue that *qi* is actually a form of highly organized information, rather in the way that a laser is a form of highly organized light. Of course skeptics deny that *qi* is anything more than a quaint idea, like the belief in unicorns, say, or an honest politician. Part of our Western skepticism derives from the fact that *qi* either as a force or substance or both (interestingly, light is both energy and substance, wave and particle) hasn't been identified, measured, or controlled in a lab to anyone's satisfaction, and here in the West, if it can't be probed in a lab, usually with plenty of expensive electronics, then it's hardly worthy of discussion (before we had the tools to measure and manipulate electromagnetism, remember, this force seemed just as preposterous).

This is of small concern to the millions of practitioners of traditional Chinese medicine and their patients, or to martial artists, however. As they have for thousands of years, these men and women are making good use of *qi*, either as an organizing concept for their practice, or as a quite real force or substance that can be manipulated to treat disease and promote health and longevity.

In Chinese medicine, ill health is thought to occur when the flow of *qi* is stagnant, blocked, or out of balance, and thus the practitioner's aim is to alter or increase the flow of *qi*, with acupuncture, acupressure, massage, herbal remedies, diet changes, and practices such as *Yoga, Qigong, Taijiquan*, or *Yiquan*.

These disciplines also place much more responsibility for health on the patient, thus it's up to the patient to supplement treatments with daily practice of the appropriate exercises. Indeed, the internal cultivation of the life force is paramount; the health practitioner may apply external modalities like acupuncture to help promote a cure, but true health is possible only when the patient has actively worked to develop his or her own *qi*, a process that involves not just physical, but mental and spiritual transformation.

This approach to medicine is fundamentally different from our Western approach, in which a largely passive patient is acted on; the patient's responsibility here is usually limited to remembering to take the appropriate pills at the appropriate times, to showing up at appointments on time, and of course to paying his bills. These Eastern disciplines are thus excellent models for us here and now as we try to take control of our own lives and change our life habits to promote our own health and longevity in an era of declining health care resources and rising costs.

When it comes to aging in particular, disciplines such as *Yiquan* might be especially important. Aging can be seen ultimately as a decline in the life force or vitality, with death the endpoint of this decline, and since disciplines like *Yiquan* work directly to cultivate vitality, then they might well prove to be among the most valuable resources available to us as we strive for the longest, most vital lives possible.

In any case, I can assure you that as you practice *Yiquan*, you will confirm in your own life the reality of *qi*. You won't have to depend on anyone to tell you it exists, or that it doesn't. That's all that matters.

Yi

How to define *yi* presents even more difficult problems. Philosophers have from the beginning of human civilization wondered what is consciousness, whether it's the ordinary everyday consciousness, the awareness, say, of a bug on the wall, or some sort of universal consciousness that permeates all of what we think of reality, or rather the refined, focused consciousness we mean when we talk about *yi*. Or perhaps all of the above.

In the internal martial arts, classical teaching has it that the *qi* follows *yi*. That is, the *qi* goes where the mind directs, and in practice, they are inseparable. That's simple enough to understand, in theory. And yet most internal disciplines don't directly go about training the mind in a systematic way to focus and concentrate consciousness, and most writings on the

18

matter don't have much to say about what is the mind, let alone how to train it. Thus I believe that *Yiquan* represents the latest step in the evolution of these internal disciplines. I believe that too many students of the internal arts go about developing their *qi* and they become quite accomplished in this, but they neglect the role of focused intention. Their bodies fill with *qi*, which is fine, but they lack the refined ability to direct or shape that *qi*, either internally or externally.

The consciousness or intention (and we all tend to use the terms interchangeably) I speak of here when I talk about *yi* is not everyday consciousness. It's special, and comes from practice and the clear intention to develop it. In a sense, refined intention comes from intention; you need the idea first, the goal, and this then informs and gives shape to your practice. It's a particular attitude to practice, and it makes all the difference. You can practice *zhanzhuang* or *Taijiquan* or *Qigong* every day for years, but if you don't have a specific concept in mind as you practice — in our case *yi* — you won't get everything you can out of it.

In *Zen* and some other philosophies of enlightenment, people talk of "mindfulness," a special attention to the moment that involves body, mind, and spirit. It's concentration, but concentration without becoming so attached to the moment that you lose sight of what's going on around you. This gets at the sort of mental state we mean when we talk about *yi*. *Yi* unites body, mind, and spirit in the moment; it's an arousal, but relaxed. It can yield enormous power, but it is gentle and sensitive. While it is consciousness, it isn't a dictatorial consciousness that is out to produce results. *Yi* is both intent and letting go, direction and release. In combat, it's being "in" the moment, but relaxed and able to respond appropriately and instantly to whatever comes its way, without having to sort through a lot of preconceived notions, techniques, or habit patterns.

Yiquan will seem very much like meditation to anyone who has had experience with that practice. In truth, *Yiquan* and meditation are very similar in many regards, including principles of breathing and posture. They have somewhat similar goals, too, though not entirely. Meditators are seeking relaxation and calmness at one level, and at a loftier level, a particular state of consciousness or enlightenment, a sense of one's place as part of all existence.

Yiquan has rather more mundane goals: the cultivation of *qi* for improved health; a greater ability to focus *yi* while maintaining a state of relaxed alertness and readiness; and finally the "unlearning" of old habits of posture and movements and a fuller integration of body and mind. Of course, enlightenment is always welcome. ■

Yiquan in Action

Exactly what is *Yiquan*, then? It's a method of unfolding human potential, but a method that's not shackled by tradition or established, rigid ways of doing things. Rather, it's a system guided by a few fundamental principles. External techniques are unimportant. They're like songs you learn. What's important when you learn a song? The words? Or the quality of your voice and the feeling with which you sing? Your *qi*, directed by your *yi*, is like a singer's voice. If you have *yi* and *qi*, you can do anything.

The three simple aspects of *Yiquan* are sitting, standing and movement. Movement in our practice includes moving the body slowly and gently while remaining grounded in your central equilibrium, and more vigorous movement as in push hands.

Because movement begins in stillness, our practice begins with sitting, and from sitting to standing, or *zhanzhuang* — standing foundation — the centerpiece of *Yiquan*, and the focus of this volume.

Zhanzhuang is the most effective practice for cultivating the flow of *qi* through the body. *Zhanzhuang* reveals where there's tension, where the flow of *qi* is blocked, the breath constricted. As you relax, your *qi* will flow naturally to points of weakness to begin the process of healing and rejuvenation. The most important thing is that you feel comfortable. These sensations are called "experiencing *qi*."

As the *qi* begins to flow more freely, you will feel more deeply relaxed. You'll raise your hands and begin the process of circulating the *qi* through the meridians. There are several different positions in *zhanzhuang*, each of which is intended to direct *qi* to various parts of the body and internal organs, according to principles of traditional Chinese medicine. Here, we'll introduce just a few of them, as a foundation for further practice and development.

While some systems work to develop the *qi* or internal energy, and other practices such as meditation seek to develop among other things one's *yi* or mental focus, *Yiquan* creates an environment in which each of us can develop both *qi* and *yi* together; think of the *qi* as the "raw materials", and the *yi* as the blueprint or instructions for using those materials. Both must be present for optimal health and function.

The practice is based on the "Three Harmonies":

• Harmonize your body: Put your body in a comfortable position.
• Harmonize your breath: Breathe normally without any effort to control or manipulate its flow.
• Harmonize your mind: Be here and now. You may find yourself daydreaming, or thinking about work or other matters. When this happens, simply let the thoughts go and return to the here and now.

This practice is especially valuable for older men and women, or anyone troubled by injury or disease, since it specifically helps improve and maintain balance, flexibility, and strength. It's an excellent form of exercise, since it has as a specific intent both increased vitality and improved longevity. I think such practice is good for everyone, and particularly important in helping to slow aging, and preserve vitality and independence, even in the very old.

Wear loose, comfortable clothing. Pleasant surroundings help, a quiet spot in the park, perhaps under a tree. Indoors, your room should be light and well-ventilated, but free of drafts. The only equipment you'll need is a sturdy chair that is the proper height for you, so that when you sit on it, your upper and lower legs form a 90-degree or right angle.

These positions are not intended to be practiced for strength. In this approach, strength comes from a state of relaxation. Rather than "muscle," *qi* "fills" your limbs, so they become both strong and supple.

You don't need to practice these in the order presented here. Let your feeling be your guide. If you feel like starting out in second position or third position, do so. If you feel like standing in second position for 30 minutes or an hour, do so. But don't force yourself into any position or to hold any position if it makes you tense or uncomfortable. The goal here is to let your *qi* flow freely, and you can't do that if you are tight or feeling uncomfortable. The following are laid out in the order in which they are normally practiced by beginners. But again, it's quite OK to change the sequence or otherwise vary the routine to suit what feels best.

Sitting

Sit on the edge of a sturdy chair so that your upper and lower legs, and upper body and legs form right angles.

• Your feet should rest flat on the floor, parallel and about shoulder width apart.

• Rest your hands lightly on your thighs. Relax your shoulders.

• As you sit, gently push the top and back of your head up toward the sky to stretch your spinal column. Imagine that there's a filament of energy running from the base of your spine, up your spine, and through your head, and that your entire spinal column is stretching upwards along this filament, that it is gently pulling upwards. As you sit, now and then remind yourself of this filament or line gently pulling up on your spinal column and head.

• With your eyes level, gaze off into the distance without focusing on anything in particular for a moment. Then close your eyes.

• At this point, your awareness is probably located behind your eyes. A fundamental principle of this practice is that your *qi* tends to concentrate where your awareness is. Now you want to "sink your *qi*" by letting your awareness sink down to your *dantian* (*tan tien*), a point about two inches below your navel, thought in Chinese medicine to be the center of the storage of *qi*.

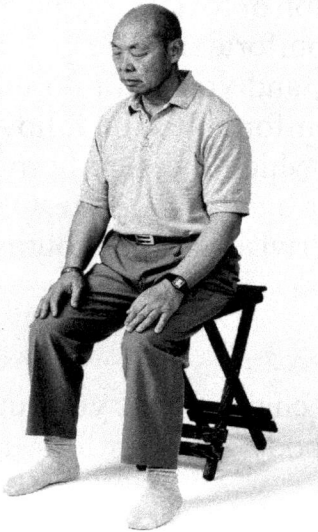

• Breathe regularly and slowly, and of most importance, breathe naturally. Let thoughts

24

come and go. Don't try to think. And don't try not to think. As thoughts come, as they will, don't dwell on them or grasp at them. Simply acknowledge the thoughts and then return your awareness to the *dantian*.

The goal at this point is a quality called *song* in Chinese. Loosely translated, it means relaxation (literally "let go"), but this is a special type of relaxation. We generally think of relaxation as a diminishing of consciousness and decreasing physical activity. But *song* is a relaxed state of alertness and readiness. Imagine a cat seemingly asleep in the sun, its eyes closed to mere slits. It's totally relaxed, but ready to pounce. This is *song*.

Practice this sitting posture for five or ten minutes, or as long as you want. When you feel like it, stand.

Standing (zhanzhuang)

Standing is the heart of this practice. It is while standing that you will learn to integrate the upper and lower body, the right and left sides of your body, and front and back, developing a clear sense of your own center in relation to gravity. It seems simple enough, of course. What could be simpler than standing? But this is standing with a particular purpose.

The theory underlying this practice is that our bodies can become "dis-integrated" by the strains of daily living. Through the alignment of the body in the most relaxed relation with gravity, the development of the relaxed readiness of *song,* and the development of the ability to concentrate or direct awareness, body and mind become more fully integrated. At the same time, this practice helps cultivate *qi*, which flows with increasing abundance throughout the body. This practice is based on the notion that disease and premature mortality occur when the *qi* is blocked or constricted. This practice aids in the development of abundant *qi*, and then the freer flowing of *qi* throughout the body. The first posture is called the *wuji* (void) posture:

• Stand slowly. Your feet should still be shoulder width and parallel. Bend your knees just slightly, so they are not locked. Next, tuck your pelvis under slightly to flatten the inward curve of the small of your back. Let your hands hang relaxed at your sides. Your head should be upright, your spine elongated along that filament of energy we mentioned above. Your weight should be shifted slightly forward, toward the balls of your feet (the *yongquan* or "bubbling well," as it's called), not back on your heels.

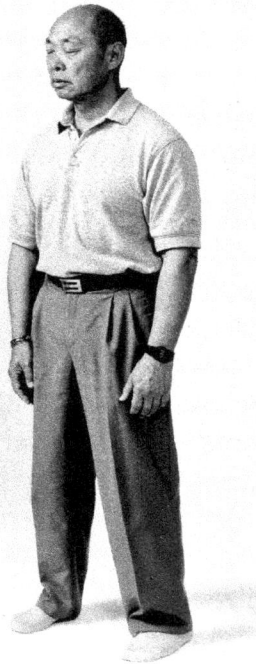

• Continue to breathe as before, with your awareness on your *dantian*. As with sitting, now and then "play" with your awareness, but then let your awareness return to your *dantian*.

• Whenever you feel uncomfortable, sit down for a few moments, again maintaining the same state of *song*, or relaxed readiness, your awareness located in

Wuji Posture

your *dantian*. It's very important not to force yourself to stand or hold any posture to the point you become uncomfortable and tense. The *qi* can't flow where the muscles are tight.

Practice the *wuji* posture, with sitting as needed, for 20 to 30 minutes, or longer if you are able. You will want to stand longer once you are in touch with your "comfort zone."

After a few days of *wuji* practice, as your *qi* begins to flow more freely, you may find yourself experiencing unusual sensations as the *qi* begins to work through blocks. Your hands may feel warm or cold. You may feel the urge to move slowly, twisting from side to side, or raising your arms, but without conscious effort, as if they're floating up. Go ahead, give in to it. Some may begin to shake as the *qi* works through blocks. Others may experience a variety of emotions, from joy to anger to sadness. That's normal. Let it happen. Let the feelings and sensations come and go as they will. Acknowledge them, but try not to become attached. When you find yourself dwelling on an emotion, thought, or sensation, take a deep breath and sink your awareness back to your *dantian*.

Master Wang also identified several characteristic sensations associated with this practice that mark a transition into later or more accomplished stages of practice. Many of these characteristic sensations will seem almost contradictory at first, until you've experienced them — all of the theory underlying *Yiquan* is eventually confirmed by personal, physical experience. These include a sense of lightness, but also of fullness; a sense of solidness, almost as if you are a statue cast of metal and rooted to the ground, but of agility and quickness at the same time. As you cultivate your *qi* and it works through blocks to flow freely throughout your body, it seems almost as if you're being filled with air, like a tire... the air is light, almost "nothing," and yet the tire is incredibly tough.

Since *qi* tends to follow awareness, you might be tempted to put your awareness at the sites of blocks or injuries, where you need particular healing. That's okay, but it should come later in your practice. For now, try to keep your awareness focused on your *dantian*. This is because *qi* naturally flows where it's needed; the body possess it's own innate wisdom, and will heal itself, if left to itself. If you keep your awareness on your *dantian*, your *qi* will eventually "overflow" from there, and flow naturally to those points where it is most needed, without benefit of diagnosis or your meddling. The problem with literally directing your *qi* is that you may not know where it's needed most. Your body does.

• Now and then, "check in" on your posture. Is your pelvis tucked under? Are your knees slightly bent? Is your weight over the balls of your feet? Are you relaxed?

There are eight different positions in *zhanzhuang* following the *wuji* position. Each position, as noted above, is intended to direct *qi* to various parts of the body and internal organs, according to the principles of traditional Chinese medicine. These positions also help develop a stable and strong stance.

First Position

This is the basis for a number of other positions, and it begins to bring us more closely to the realm of the martial arts.

When you feel relaxed, raise your arms slowly to shoulder level. Imagine that you aren't raising them, but rather that they are floating up, that you are holding a large beach ball, which fills and lifts your arms.

Imagine with each inhalation and exhalation that a ball of energy centered in your *dantian* expands and contracts against your hands. Imagination is an important part of *Yiquan* practice. It is in the stillness of *zhanzhuang* that what is at first imaginary becomes manifest as reality. The human nervous system does not make clear distinctions between what is imagined and what is real (that distinction in itself may be in error), thus what we imagine, in the quiet state of *zhanzhuang*, can powerfully influence our physical reality.

• Hold your arms as if they are wrapped around that beach ball. Your hands should be relaxed, the fingers slightly spread. There should be no sharp angles in your shoulders, elbows or wrists — *qi* doesn't flow easily around sharp angles.

• Your hands should be spread apart about the width of your shoulders or perhaps a bit less.

• As ever, your awareness should be

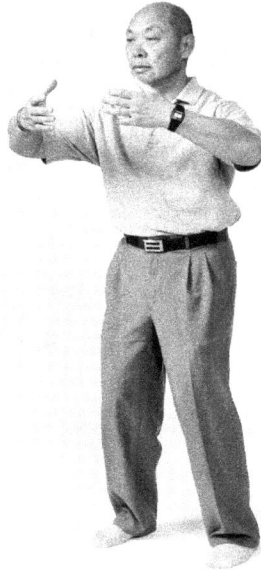

First Position

29

located in your *dantian*. However, now and then "play" with your awareness; move it to other areas of the body.

• Breathe deeply and evenly. If you find yourself daydreaming, let your thoughts come and go, without clinging to any of them.

• Don't hold this position so long that you tighten. In the beginning, you may be able to hold this position only a moment or two. When you feel tense, take a few deep breaths as you imagine the tension draining down and out the bottoms of your feet. If that doesn't work, then return to *wuji* position, or sitting, or move on to the second position.

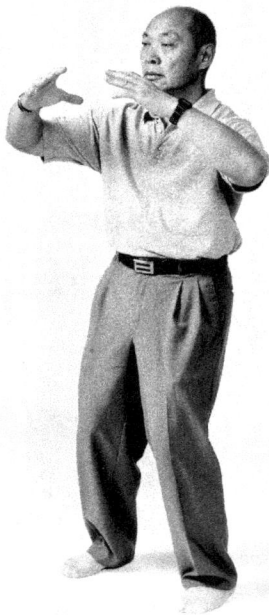

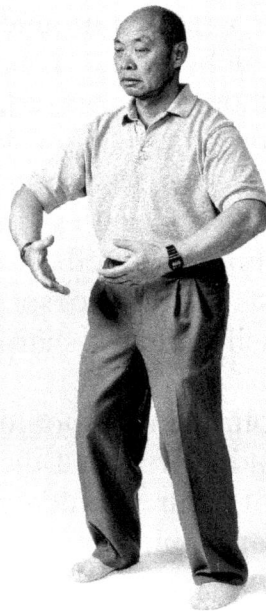

Second Position   **Third Position**

Second Position

Maintaining the same posture, rotate your palms so they face downward. Be sure that you remain relaxed, and that you are still "holding that beach ball," now with your hands on top.

Third Position

Still "holding the beach ball," rotate your arms down around it, until your hands are at about the level of your *dantian*. Your palms now should be facing slightly upwards. Your fingers are still slightly spread, but relaxed. All of the basic principles of posture, breathing and awareness still apply.

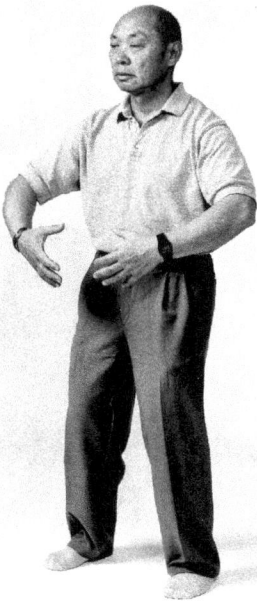

Fourth Position

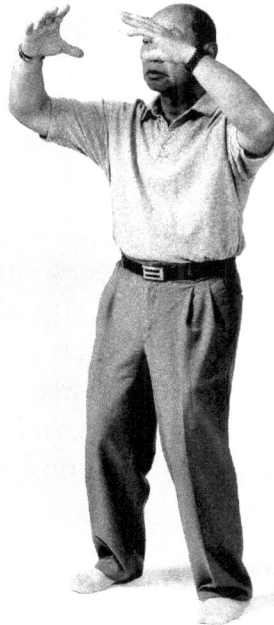

Fifth Position

31

Fourth Position

The difference between third and fourth positions is a small one. Simply rotate your hands toward you, so your palms now face your *dantian*.

Fifth Position

Inhale, and let your arms rise, as if floating upwards, until your hands are at the level of your eyebrows, your palms facing down. Again, imagine that your arms are light and filled with *qi*, that it takes no effort to hold them here. If you find yourself growing tense, lower your hands to *wuji* position and rest until the tension eases.

Sixth Position

From the fifth position, slowly lower and straighten your arms to about the level of your shoulders. Slightly extend your fingers. Imagine that your *qi* is flowing out through your arms, along your fingers, and out the tips. Sink slightly. Remember to keep your pelvis tucked under. If you feel uncomfortable, return to the *wuji* posture or sitting.

Seventh Position

Lower your arms slowly

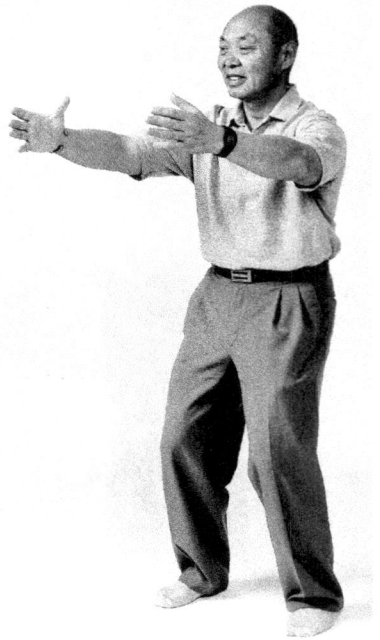

Sixth Position

32

and at the same time, turn your palms down. Your hands should now be at the level of your waist. Imagine that you are standing in waist-deep water and that your hands are floating on the water.

Sink slightly and relax. With each exhalation, feel any tension settling down out of your body through the bottoms of your feet. Again, if you feel tense, return to the *wuji* posture or sitting.

Eighth Position
To move from the seventh position to the eighth, imagine that the water on which your hands were floating is draining out, and your hands are sinking, until they are almost — but not quite — by your thighs, almost as in the *wuji* posture. Here, however,

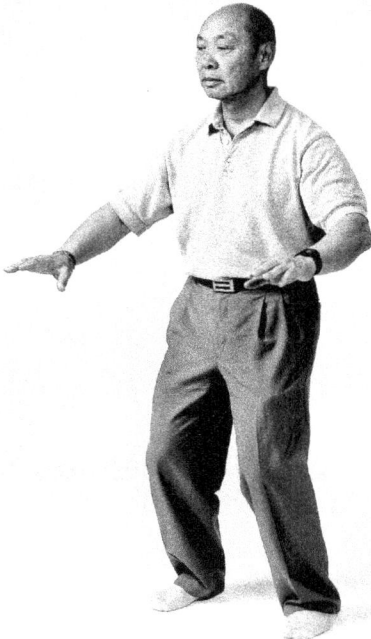

Seventh Position   **Eighth Position**

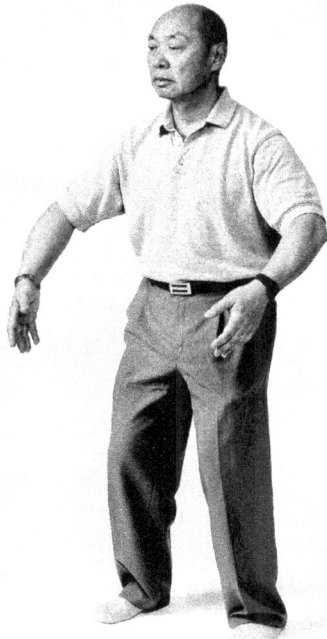

your hands are held away from your body just slightly, the fingers pointing down and extended as in the sixth position. With each exhalation, imagine your *qi* flowing down your arms and out the tips of your fingers. As you inhale, imagine the *qi* returning.

"Half squat"

This is a transitional exercise that provides a bridge between stillness and movement. It's great for strengthening the legs and all the joints. When you feel rested, return to the seventh position, your palms turned toward the floor, your hands at the level of your abdomen.

Your feet should still be shoulder width and parallel, your weight shifted slightly toward the balls of your feet, your pelvis tucked under, your posture upright. Now, begin:

• Exhale, and as you do so, sink slightly, bending your knees and lowering your hands to just below your waist. Imagine your hands are floating on water, and that the water level has dropped.

• Inhale, and as you do so, rise slightly, raising your hands back to the level of your *dantian*, or a bit higher. Imagine, again, that the water has risen, carrying your hands with it.

In this exercise, feel free to play with your awareness. When you exhale, let your awareness sink down your legs through your feet into the earth. When you inhale, let your awareness travel back up your legs, through your *dantian*, up your spine, through the top of your head and toward the sky.

There are refinements of this particular "awareness play" involving the direction of awareness down the front of the body, and up the back, but the basic routine described here will suffice. In later volumes, We'll discuss these more directed forms of awareness play. ■

Some Thoughts
on Empty Force *(Kongjing)*

I said earlier I think too much emphasis on the development and use of *kongjing* or empty force is a distraction from the true spirit of *Yiquan*. After having learned the technique myself and confirmed that empty force is quite real, and after having taught the technique to many of my students, I must say that I now believe there is nothing miraculous about it. Empty force is simply an extension of well-developed awareness, what is sometimes called "super listening *qi*," an intensified field of biomagnetism. We all have energy fields around our bodies, whether we're trained or untrained. For example, think how you may know when someone is looking at you, though your back is turned. This is a rudimentary type of empty force. It's a sixth sense that we all have in varying degrees, a sense that can be developed.

I first encountered *kongjing* on my first trip back to China in 1979, when I went to visit Cai *Sifu*. I saw him working with his students, not touching them, but using *kongjing*, his "empty force." They would jump back 20 to 30 feet when he merely pointed at them.

At first, I could hardly believe my eyes, figuring it had to be either a miracle or a joke. But in discussing it with Cai later, he explained that they were merely playing with the intention and its perception. In other words, with subtle energy, not irresistible force.

Cai has never claimed, and would never claim, that his empty force is irresistible. Whenever questioned, he is quite clear on the fact that this is a perceptual game for the training of awareness, that there is no magic at work.

What is developed in this training is a very special type of awareness and sensitivity; I think of this as "intentional awareness."

As your *qi* develops, your field of energy strengthens and widens. And with practice it's possible to shape and focus and direct this field toward others. Moreover, as you become more accomplished in this, you become more sensitive to the energy fields of others. Indeed, this increased sensitivity to others is, I believe, the primary importance of empty force.

Some practitioners of *kongjing* focus on the use of *kongjing* from a distance, never touching the other person. Cai *Sifu* and his students practiced both from a distance, and touching the other person in push hands exercises. As one develops *kongjing*, one becomes more sensitive to the other's intention. The point of contact becomes the gate of access to the opponent's center, and to control over it.

It was certainly an effective type of training, as I came to understand when I played push hands with Cai's students. They were so sensitive and quick that at that time I could not push them. They perceived and were able to neutralize my intention to push them at the very moment I had it. That was a real eye opener.

Practice in empty force, when done in the right spirit, should teach us to listen better to others, literally, of course, but also in terms of another's energy field, so you sense from the other's energy what the other is going to do before he or she does it. In *Yiquan* practice, quite often we will "play" with empty force, where one sends, the other receives. With such practice, the sender and receiver become more skilled and their sensitivities to one another increase. Empty force is a type of communication, in other words, and a very powerful type of communication.

And like any form of communication, it can be used for good or ill; used correctly, it can create peace and harmony. ∎

A Few Terms and Names

The *pinyin* spelling of the terms and names below is based on the Mandarin pronunciation, with a few exceptions. The characters are mostly the simplified versions.

Bāguàzhǎng (八卦掌): Literally "eight trigram palm," referring to the trigrams of the *I Ching* (*Book of Changes*). It's one of the main internal arts, along with *Taijiquan* and *Xingyiquan*. Practice involves circular movements.

Cài Sōngfāng (蔡松芳) (1931-): Cai *Sifu*'s name is pronounced "Choi" in Cantonese, but it's usually spelled "Cai" in English-language publications, thus that spelling here. Cai is Fong's very good friend from Shanghai. He's one of China's most renowned *Qigong* masters. It was while working with Cai that Fong first encountered "empty force," or *kongjing*, in practice.

dāntián (丹田): A set of three regions in your body that serve as dynamic storage points for *qi*, rather like the crests of waves in river rapids that store energy. The lower *dantian* is the one that gets the most attention in the martial arts, especially the internal arts. It's about three finger widths below the navel and two behind it. The middle *dantian* is at the level of the heart. The upper *dantian* is in the forehead, roughly between the eyebrows.

Dào (道): Variously translated as "way," "path," "route," "road," or more loosely as "doctrine" or "principle." In the *Dao De Jing* (*Tao Te Ching*) by Laozi (Lao Tsu), the first two lines of the first verse tell us that "the Dao that is called Dao is not the Dao. Names can name no lasting name." That is, while all things come from the *Dao,* the *Dao* is beyond description by language and logic, meaning that to understand the *Dao*, one must go past language and logic to access that internal reservoir of unspoken wisdom within each of us.

Dǒng Yīngjíe (董英杰) (1898-1961): Fong Ha's first teacher in the Yang style of *Taijiquan*. Dong was born in Hebei, China, a senior student of Yang Chengfu. He wrote a book titled *T'ai chi ch'uan Explained* or, variously, *Principles of T'ai chi ch'uan*, first published in 1948.

Gōngfū (功夫): Literally "skill" (*gong*) and "man" (*fu*): Achievement in a technique or skill, a general term for many types of martial arts.

Hàn Xīngyùan (韓星垣) (1915-1983): A.k.a. Ruoshui, Han was born in Hebei Province. He first learned *Xingyiquan* from his father. Later, he studied with Wang Xiangzhai. It was Han who introduced Fong to the power of *zhanzhuang*.

kōngjīng (空勁): Literally "empty force." An extension of well-developed awareness, sometimes called "super listening *qi*." As your *qi* develops through practices such as *Yiquan* and *Qigong*, the field of energy in and around your body strengthens and expands. With practice, it becomes possible to focus and direct this field toward others, as you become more sensitive to another's energy field. In *Yiquan* practice, we often "play" with empty force, where one sends and the other receives. Think of empty force as a special type of communication.

nèigōng (內功): The cultivation of innate abilities and potential. The term refers to a variety of breathing, meditation, and spiritual practices associated with *Daoism* and the internal martial arts.

qì (氣): A "subtle energy" that flows through the body, closely related to physical, mental, and spiritual health. It's variously translated as "life force," "breath," "universal energy," or "human energy field," though none of these translations quite captures the true meaning of the term. (See also *ki*, *prana*; possibly also the Greek *pneuma*). *Qi* follows *yi* (see below).

Qìgōng (氣功): Literally "energy practice." *Yiquan*, "intention practice," is a form of *Qigong*, but with more emphasis on the role of the mind in the development of *qi*, healing, and of course the martial arts.

quán (拳): System, practice, or boxing.

shén (神): Soul, spiritual or mental energy.

Sīfù (师傅) (a.k.a. *shifu* in Mandarin): Honored or skillful teacher or tutor.

sōng (松): Loosely, a state of minimum tension in the physical body and abandonment of attachment in the mind. Actions taken while in this state are highly efficient and allow exceptional coordination of integrated movements.

Tàijíquán (太极拳): Literally "Great Ultimate Boxing" (*quan*: fist or boxing). Though a martial art, it's also practiced for a variety of reasons, including improved health and longevity, and as a form of meditation. There are several styles of *Taijiquan*, including the Yang style.

Wáng Xīangzhāi (王芗斋) (1885-1963): Born in Hebei Province, founder of the *Yiquan* system.

wújí (无极): Lacking a highest point, ultimate, boundless, infinite. Wuji can be thought of as a neutral state with no separation into *yin* or *yang* at the highest level. *Yin* and *yang* here refer to the correspondences of seeming opposites such as soft and hard, passive and active, etc., which are in fact complementary aspects of the whole. See also *wuwei* (无为) a concept meaning non-action, non-doing, or non-forcing, an important concept in *Daoism*. If one is in total harmony with the *Dao*, one behaves in completely natural way.

Xīngyìquán (形意拳): Form and mind practice, or "boxing." *Xing* is the manifestation of the intention (*yi*) for guiding and controlling the body and is an important concept in empty force. *Xing* also has an emotional element in this context; it describes an internal spirit that underlies any plan, one's resilience and optimism and willingness to carry on.

Yáng Chéngfǔ (杨澄甫) (1883-1936): Yang Luchan's grandson. Yang Chengfu is the author of two books on the Yang style, *Application Methods of Taijiquan*, published in 1931, and *Essence and Applications of Taijiquan*, published in 1934. His second book was translated into English in 2005.

Yáng Lùchán (杨露禅) (1799-1872): The founder of the Yang style of Taijiquan.

Yáng Shǒuzhōng (1910-1985) (杨守中): A.k.a. Yang Zhenming, Yang Chengfu's eldest son. After Dong Yingjie's death, Fong continued to study with Yang Shouzhong.

yì (意): Mind, intention, desire, wanting, also "consciousness." *Yi* is clear intellect, the conception and execution of a plan. The clearer your *yi*, the better the execution of the plan.

Yìquán (意拳): Intention practice, or "boxing," development of one's *yi* and *qi*. Also known as "*Dachengquan*," which means "great achievement boxing," but Wang Xiangzhai felt that was a bit too grandiose, and, having mastered *Xingyiquan*, and having reduced his own practice to the basics, he dropped the "*xing*" and thus we now have *Yiquan*.

yǒngquán (涌泉): The "bubbling well," an acupuncture point in the crease between the big toe and the side of foot both sideways and lengthwise. It is the preferred point of ground contact while standing.

zhànzhūang (站桩): *Zhan* (stand) and *zhuang* (pillar or foundation), the heart of *Yiquan*. *Zhanzhuang* is the most effective practice for cultivating the flow of *qi* through the body. *Zhanzhuang* reveals where there's tension, where the flow of *qi* is blocked, the breath constricted. As you relax, your *qi* will flow naturally to points of weakness to begin the process of healing and rejuvenation. Sometimes called *wuji zhanzhuang*. ∎

Further Reading

Cai Songfang, *Wujishi Breathing Exercises from the Teachings of Cai Songfang*; Plum Publications, 2013.
>An in-depth discussion of standing breathing exercises, including the finer points of the micro- and macro-cosmic orbits and the movement of *qi* through the body. It also includes case studies of people who used *Wujishi* to cure certain illnesses and conditions.

Cheng Man-Ching, translated by Douglas Wile, *Master Cheng's Thirteen Chapters on Tai Chi Chuan*; Sweet Chi Press, 1982.
>A nice companion, from Cheng's perspective, to Tai-chi Touchstones (see below, Douglas Wile, editor).

Dong, Paul and Thomas Raffill, *Empty Force: The power of Chi for Self-defense and Energy Healing*; Blue Snake Books, 2006.
>Presumes to reveal "the secret of the empty force" and, as it says on the back cover, "how martial arts masters use its power to defend themselves against opponents without making physical contact."

Horwitz, Tem, et al, *Tai Chi Chuan, The Technique of Power*; Cloud Hands Press, 2015.
>Lots of insights clearly presented. Horwitz and his co-authors are dancers as well as scholars; they offer up a good deal of the writings of Lao Tzu, plus bits of the *I Ching*, and various other mystical and alchemical writings as a kind of philosophical support for what we do, which is sometimes handy to have, all founded on the notion that insights often begin in the flesh.

Huang Wen-Shan, *Fundamentals of Tai Chi Chuan*; South Sky Book Company, Hong Kong, 1973.

May be out of print, but used (and expensive) copies seem to be available through Amazon. It's a huge, idiosyncratic volume written in Huang's peculiar brand of English. It's hard to get through and often doesn't make a lot of sense, but it has a forward by Laura Huxley — Aldous' wife — and Huang does say right up front that "Tai Chi Ch'uan is a Chinese system of exercise or an art of life, the practice of which provides valuable help in extending man's life span, eliminating tension and increasing opportunities of physical, spiritual, and mental well-being and equilibrium." Say what you will about his prose style, you can't argue with the ideas.

Lao Tzu, *The Tao Te Ching*, edited by Lin Yutang; Modern Library, 1948.

Perhaps one of the best translations; Lin Yutang provides a discourse on each-chapter, plus relevant writings from Chuang Tzu. See in particular chapters 8, 9, 10, 15, 18, 19, 22, 24, 33, 43, 47, 48, 55, 63, 68, 69, 76 and 77. The idea is that one lives one's life according to the same principles of balance, "centeredness," mindfulness, charity, and simple commonsense that one applies (or should apply) to the practice of *Taiji*, and that the practice of *Taiji* touches all aspects of one's life by teaching these principles at "the gut level," so you know them first in the flesh and bones, not just theoretically.

Lo, Benjamin Pang Jeng, et al, *The Essence of Tai Chi Chuan, The Literary Tradition*; Blue Snake Books, 1993.

A rather more "poetic" rendition of much of what's available in Douglas Wile's *Touchstones* (see below).

Mayer, Michael, *Secrets to Living Younger Longer: The Self Healing Path of Qigong, Standing Meditation and Tai Chi*; Bodymind Healing Publications, 2007.

Michael is a psychotherapist who has studied with Fong Ha for many years. Michael notes: "One of Fong's gifts is giving his students room to interpret his transmission in their way. In this book, I put forth the way I've integrated Fong's teachings with my understanding of cross-cultural postural initiation traditions. I put forth my hypothesis that each Tai Chi movement can be looked at as having four dimensions of purpose: Self healing, spiritual unfoldment, self-defense, and finding a new life stance."

Mayer, *Bodymind Healing Psychotherapy: Ancient Pathways to Modern Health*; Bodymind Healing Publications, 2007.

Of this book, Michael writes: "My contribution to the field of psychotherapy is showing how psychotherapy is an endeavor of transforming one's life stance. Without the thousands of hours spent doing Standing Mediation Qigong through Fong's influence, my putting forth of this viewpoint would have lacked grounded depth. I showed how Qigong and the training I received from Fong could enhance an 'integral psychotherapy' by combining Qigong with traditional psychotherapies."

Mayer, *Energy Psychology: Self-healing Methods for Bodymind Health*; North Atlantic Books, 2011.

A revision of *Bodymind Healing Psychotherapy*, for a popular audience.

Mayer, *The Path of a Reluctant Metaphysician: Stories and Practices for Troubled Times*; Bodymind Healing Publications, 2012

In this book, Michael discusses how the experience of *qi* that was transmitted to him by Fong is incorporated into his Bodymind Healing approach to psychotherapy. The book speaks to the importance of having a "holistic" spiritual philosophy in this time of the "great unraveling," as Michael put it, of our personal, political, economic, cultural, and ecological world.

Shi Ming, with Siao Weijia, *Mind Over Matter: the Higher Martial Arts*; Frog Limited, 1994.
   Translated by Thomas Cleary, who does a lot of translations. An exploration of the notion of "consciousness" in the martial arts. Touches on "empty force" along the way.

Suzuki, Shunryu, *Zen Mind, Beginner's Mind*; Weatherhill, 1970.
   This has some good thoughts on the attitude one should maintain while practicing *Zazen*, and by extension, *Qigong*. *Qigong* is not necessarily *Zazen*, of course, and our goals in *Qigong* are not quite those in *Zazen* — we're after more mundane things than enlightenment, such as longevity, health and so on — but *Zazen* and *Qigong* are identical in essence, as *Zen* and *Daoism* are identical at the deepest levels.

Tang, C.S., *The Complete Book of Yiquan*; Singing Dragon, 2015.
   A comprehensive guide to the history, development, and practice of *Yiquan*. It's a big book of more than 400 pages, with a price tag to match.

Wayne, P. & Fuerst, M., *The Harvard Medical School Guide to Tai Chi*; Boston: Shamballah Publications, 2013.
   A popular yet scholarly guide to the scientific studies on *Taiji*, which reviews the scientific evidence for the healing effects of *Taiji*, which many of us took on faith when we first started practicing *Taiji* and related martial arts.

Wile, Douglas (ed.), *Tai-chi Touchstones: Yang Family Secret Transmissions*; Sweet Chi Press, 2010.

> Perhaps the best source of theory by far; most of the ideas about why we do what we do in the way we do it are contained here, though now and then somewhat obliquely. The book also offers some reasonably clear photographs showing the various techniques in use.

Wilhelm, Richard, trans., and Cary F. Baynes, *The I Ching or Book of Changes*; Bollingen Series XIX, Princeton University Press, third edition, 1969.

> This edition is the English translation of Wilhelm's German translation, which gets us a bit removed from the original text, but it could nonetheless be the best translation available. Plus it comes with a foreword by C.G. Jung himself, written in 1949 for the first edition. What's not to like? In his intro, Wilhelm writes: "The Book of Changes—*I Ching* in Chinese—is unquestionably one of the most important books in the world's literature." ∎